I0410523

Lose 50 Pounds in 50 Days!

And Keep it Off!

by

Scott S. Pribyl

Bloomington, IN  Milton Keynes, UK

authorHOUSE™

AuthorHouse™
1663 Liberty Drive, Suite 200
Bloomington, IN 47403
www.authorhouse.com
Phone: 1-800-839-8640

AuthorHouse™ UK Ltd.
500 Avebury Boulevard
Central Milton Keynes, MK9 2BE
www.authorhouse.co.uk
Phone: 08001974150

This book is a work of non-fiction. Unless otherwise noted, the author and the publisher make no explicit guarantees as to the accuracy of the information contained in this book and in some cases, names of people and places have been altered to protect their privacy.

© 2006 Scott S. Pribyl. All rights reserved.

No part of this book may be reproduced, stored in a retrieval system, or transmitted by any means without the written permission of the author.

First published by AuthorHouse 2/10/2006

ISBN: 1-4208-2163-6 (sc)

Library of Congress Control Number: 2005900448

Printed in the United States of America
Bloomington, Indiana

This book is printed on acid-free paper.

If you need to lose weight, or are tired of weighing more than you would like, please read this entire book- then, re-read it. It is brief and very concise. Not a lot of theory- just a method that I have used that has worked- for over 14 years.

At the age of 20 I weighed 196#. At age 35 I weighed 246#. In 1990, at age 35, after 50 days of trying a concept, I lost 50 pounds and again weighed 196#. Today, 2 months before my 50th birthday, I still weigh 196#.

If you want rapid weight loss, without pills, special foods, classes to attend- and want to keep it off- then read on! *(And, especially if you want to reduce your food costs!)*

Every diet I have ever tried was successful- short term- but I always put the weight back on. Sound familiar? I have synthesized a lot of different ideas I have explored into one plan that works for me- and it can work for you, too. With minimal time and little effort. Believe it.

I could expound on the many benefits of weighing less: appearance, self esteem, health, blood pressure, help with diabetes, etc. But you all know what those benefits are, already. So, let's dispense with what we all know and get right into the plan- you want results, not excessive reading. I urge everyone who wants to lose 5 to 100+ pounds to talk with your physician first. I do not recommend any stimulants or synthetic agents such as caffeine or ephedra, mua huang, etc. But, I recommend you talk to your doctor first- it's a good idea to keep your doctor informed and seek their input before you start shedding pounds

CHAPTER ONE

Start the day off right

Consider this as it works for me- 14 ½ years as of this writing: (more detail will follow in Chapters 3 and 5)

Drink a lot of "water" in the morning. 2-3 large glasses. I like flavored mineral water- many varieties, inexpensive, and no calories! Use ice and a slice of lemon to give "regular' water a better flavor. Tap water is fine, some prefer distilled. It is your choice. Once your stomach is full- with food or water- your body will indicate to you it has enough in it to start the day. Use fruit juices if you want. Or diet sodas that are caffeine free, which are better for weight reduction, in my opinion. Some people can tolerate caffeine better than others. I can't so I avoid it. My point is low, or no, calorie liquids will give you the water your body craves and give your body a "full" feeling. If you feel you need something to eat at breakfast I recommend a piece of fruit, a slice of real/true whole wheat bread, or something else very small and nutritious-after your water or fluid intake. After the water- tap,

3

distilled or mineral- you will probably not be very hungry because your body will then have what it craves and is primarily comprised of- water (and you will feel full!). Make your water taste good- be creative! It works! (Note: 2-3 large glasses, per above, means 24 to 36 ounces, total). Again, I suggest flavored mineral water

(Diet/powder drinks are Ok, but they do have calories- and milk of any sort will add further calories. Feel free to experiment, but only drink 8-16 oz., maximum, of a diet/powder drink in the morning, again, after your water- or alternate between them.)

Mid day: drink more mineral or flavored water or juice or diet drinks. Perhaps a piece of fruit or a vegetable- pickles, celery, carrots, etc. Try to avoid eating until lunch, but no/low calorie drinks are fine. I discourage coffee, however. I rarely eat lunch as I am not hungry if I drink the good tasting water drinks, diet sodas, or diet/powder drinks in the morning, at mid day, or when I might eat lunch. For lunch, if you really need food I suggest high protein foods, like meat, poultry, fish- or eggs. But not sandwiches, unless you use 1-2 slices of real/true whole wheat bread. Just the meat, poultry or fish, fairly lean, and seasoned, may be enough so you don't need bread. Depending on how much you want to lose, eat 6-12 oz. of meat, poultry or fish (tuna works well) after your water and fluids. But you probably will not be hungry after your liquids and water, and high protein foods will keep you feeling full until evening. Deviled or hard boiled eggs are great lunch snacks- again, after, your fluids, if you really need food.

Lunch: discussed above, but, again, before eating, drink 16 to 24 ounces of water, juice or diet/powder drinks- make sure you experiment and devise drinks that taste good and have low/no calories; once your stomach is full with good tasting water and fluids you probably will not be very hungry, if at all. However, if you are still hungry, (re-read the above paragraph) or, have a small portion of food- focusing on nutrition. Avoid breads (except real/true whole wheat), starches, pizza, cheese and dairy products, etc. (More will follow on food groups). After drinking the no/low calorie drinks in the quantities indicated, you won't be hungry much, if at all, anyway. I repeat this for a reason: when your stomach is full you will not want much food. If you fill your stomach with what your body craves- water, or no/low calorie drinks (that you make taste good!), and use vitamin supplements, you will have constant energy, a full feeling, needed supplemental nutrition and weight loss- all occurring in your body at the same time!

Afternoon: if you feel hungry or thirsty, again, consume 16-24 ounces of water, juice, diet drinks, etc. Diet powder/liquid drinks should be limited to 8 ounces- after you've had your other water, diet sodas, etc. More will follow on ways to make water or no/low calorie drinks taste good- it is important you enjoy the taste as you recompose your body.

Evening: Make a great tasting shake! With diet/powder drinks (for the ones I recommend please contact me), use 16-24oz. water, and

16-24 oz. of skim milk and add low calorie flavor enhancements like fat-free pudding, soy ice cream, low calorie sundae flavorings, bananas, strawberries, blueberries, and ice cubes/slivers etc. Or, if you prefer a fruitier taste, use 8 oz. water and 16 to 24 oz fruit juice (add ice also) and then add fat-free fruit gelatin, or pieces of lemon, lime, orange, apple, banana, strawberry, berries, etc. Many powdered or liquid diet drinks have flavors like chocolate, vanilla, strawberry, fudge, orange, etc. The objective here is to make a full blender- right to the top- 64 ounces, of a flavorful drink that tastes good and has low calories. I recommend vitamin supplements, with dinner, or food snacks, to insure your body has the right amounts of vitamins and minerals. (I recommend one brand in particular- contact me if you want more information on what I use and recommend.). Then, if you are still hungry, have some protein: lean meats, fish, poultry, eggs, some fats like butter, minimal cheese, nuts and vegetables. (Chapters 3 and 5 will specifically describe how to make Great tasting shakes that you will enjoy and that will fill you up!

After a 64 oz. full blender of a <u>very</u> good tasting shake, you won't be very hungry- your stomach may not be as large as what a 64 oz. blender can put into it! Think about that. Avoid fruits at dinner as well as pasta, rice, bread, etc. Starchy foods stay with me a long time and make me even hungrier. Protein rich foods keep my body full a long time. (More about making these foods very good to eat will follow- trust me, the contents of this book will help you lose weight while you give your body what it needs, with very good tasting food- and a full feeling, with no need to feel hungry). You will, as you can imagine, need to urinate more than you may now, but remember what your body is primarily compromised of? That's right, water.

As you can imagine, by consuming the amounts of liquids I've listed above- which I only recommend until you've reached your goal weight, then you can cut back- unless you like the liquids- (but make the liquids fun and enjoyable!) I recommend 100+ ounces per day, during the day, of various liquids until you have reached your goal weight. I still consume 64-80 ounces per day. I still do this and maintain my weight. When I go back to more food, especially starchy foods and fruits, I can gain weight- so I increase the water and liquids until I am back to my weight goal. This plan has worked for me- it can work for you as long as you utilize it. Yes, we want immediate weight loss, but the goal is to keep it off permanently. (And not be hungry and have plenty of energy!)

If you feel the need for a late night snack- which does not occur often if you've had a fair amount of protein rich food for dinner (if you even need that), try nuts, or a little cheese. Microwave popcorn can be good before bed- an hour before- but starchy foods can cause later hunger. Protein rich foods seem to keep the stomach and body feeling full.

Now, this is a day that started off right and ended right. Be careful not to have your evening shake too close to your bedtime. Try to allow 4-5 hours before bedtime, and stop the liquids at that time. You want a full night's sleep without waking for bathroom trips more than once or twice. And, don't forget your vitamin and mineral supplements with your dinner shake or food. My energy is more than ample to perform a demanding job that is 50 hours per week by day, and I exert a lot of effort and energy in my hobby. A good night's sleep is very important. Stop the liquids 4-5 hours before bedtime and you'll feel fine when you awake in the morning. (By that time, 100+ ounces will be all you need or probably want- until the next day when your body will begin to let you know it is craving more water and liquids). Don't be surprised if you need <u>less</u> sleep and have <u>more</u> energy as you lose weight!

CHAPTER 2
Food Choices

Who has time to calculate every calorie or gram of protein, fat or carbohydrate a given food will have? Try this instead:

***After** you've had your water and liquids for a given "meal":*

Foods to avoid:

Starchy foods, like potatoes, processed breads, pasta, rice, chips, too much popcorn, grains. Too much sugar, cereal, and other processed grains will hurt your progress. Once you've hit your weight goal, add some of these foods if you'd like. I caution you though: these foods leave me feeling full and a bit uncomfortable, and I later get hungry. They have never helped me lose weight- except a little popcorn on occasion (or a slice of whole wheat/grain bread). Just use these foods sparingly until you've hit your goal.

Fruit: of course, some fruit is good. I only speak from experience, but too much fruit does not make me feel full and I get hungrier afterward.

Keep the fruit intake low until you've reached your goal weight.

Fats: too much cheese, milk, ice cream, creamed sauces, etc. will add calories, and will not make you feel full. You may get even hungrier. Use these foods in limited amounts until you have reached your goal. I mention "reaching your goal" often and there is a reason, which will follow.

Excessive amounts of vegetables: during your weight loss period, too many vegetables may leave you feeling hungrier and hungrier. Use vegetables, but after you have had your water and fluids, and eaten your high protein foods. You want to eat foods that taste good, do good things for you and keep you feeling full. Too many vegetables during the weight loss period can hinder your progress. Once you've reached your weight goal, I recommend a lot of great tasting vegetables (Chapter 5).

Liquids to avoid:

Regular soda, too much fruit juice (high calorie and sugar content), excessive alcohol (I allow myself 6-8 beers per week- usually on weekends). In the beginning you may want to eliminate alcohol or limit your intake to a "few" per week. I avoid milk except skim for making great tasting shakes. I think drinks that add electrolytes, but are low in calories, are OK in moderation- but the sodium content is a concern. Only drink 3-5 of these drinks per week, maximum, and make sure you drink a lot of water (sound familiar?) to flush your system. Coffee is something I avoid for a host of reasons. I can not encourage it.

Foods that will help:

High protein foods like meats, poultry, fish/tuna, etc. Fairly lean. Eggs are good also. These foods leave me feeling full and give me plenty of energy. However, if you have high cholesterol or diabetes concerns, stay in touch with your doctor as these foods might elevate same. My belief is high protein foods eaten in larger amounts than usual, for a short period of time, if I am losing weight, help me. Once your weight goal is achieved balance your diet accordingly.

Vegetables: after I have had my liquids and evening shake, I might- if I am still hungry, have a high protein food, say 6-10 oz. of beef or poultry, or up to 16 oz. of baked or broiled fish or tuna. By that time, my stomach is beyond full and this combination leaves me full a very long time!. If I want a bit more food, or as a late snack or during the day, 8 to 16 oz. of vegetables is good and helpful. More will follow on how to make those vegetables taste very, very good. (However, when I consume 100+ oz. of water and liquids I rarely have any hunger for much food- try it).

Fruits: 1 piece a day is all I recommend until you've reached your goal. If that.

Nuts: preferably with no, or minimal salt. They make me feel full and taste good. A cup or two during the day, if you are hungry, is a good idea-unless you have allergies to certain nuts.

Salads: 1 a day, if you'd like, after high protein food and after liquids. Eat more upon achieving your desired weight- if you like salad.

So, what do I do on a given week day: I drink the water as outlined in chapter 1- mainly flavored mineral water with ice. Tastes great and is very refreshing- a slice of lemon, lime or orange is even better! Sometimes I will have a diet/powder drink during the day- but usually not. Most such drinks are composed of water primarily, anyway. If I drink 24 to 48 oz. of mineral water or juice combination in the morning I take small amounts of vitamins/minerals. This does not upset my stomach at all as the water has filled my stomach and the vitamins seem to release easily. Experiment with supplements- if you <u>need</u> a little food, eat 1 piece of fruit, or some nuts, or a vegetable serving- after your liquids. Or, an egg or two. (I do not tolerate high fat meats well, so I avoid them. Same with fried foods).

If I drink 24 to 48 oz. of water, juice, diet soda, no/low calorie diet/powder drinks during the morning I usually am not hungry by lunch time. I do not have a mid morning snack because the liquids for breakfast have me still feeling full and with plenty of energy. For lunch, if I truly am hungry, I drink the liquids and add some nuts, or lean meat or chicken, or vegetables. Occasionally, an apple, orange or banana. That normally tides me over until dinner. (But I rarely eat lunch as I am just not hungry if I drink good fluids). If I want something mid afternoon I drink 16-20 oz. of diet soda, again, with no caffeine, or mineral water. I suggest taking water with you to work or wherever you go. But: make sure you make it taste good! Give it some flavor! Add a slice of fruit, or...............use your imagination. (Or, look at what I use in Chapter 5).

For dinner I have had the best results with the full blender, 64 oz. I mentioned, of a powdered shake- flavored as I want it, so that it tastes really good and fills me up. With so many ways to flavor these drinks, that utilize minimal calories, I look forward to that huge refreshing drink. I take my vitamin and mineral supplements at that time as my stomach is very full. If I am still hungry I will eat some meat, poultry, fish, tuna, eggs, etc.; or have 8 to 16 oz. of vegetables. But with 64 oz. of a great tasting shake in my stomach, I am rarely hungry. Lately, I have been eating more meat and vegetables and just having water for my dinner. Either method seems to work just fine- once my weight goal has been realized.

For a late night snack, <u>if</u> I still am hungry, I eat nuts, or deviled eggs, or a salad, sometimes microwave popcorn. I stop drinking liquids 4-5 hours before bedtime- when possible- so I don't have more than 1-2 bathroom trips during the night. I practice what I preach. I have had high blood pressure since 1982, age 27; the best thing I can do is keep my weight down and not eat starchy foods.

Chapter 3

How to make these liquids and foods taste great!

(And keep your food costs lower!)

Water: use a slice of fruit and ice. Try tap or distilled; I prefer flavored mineral water- a lot of it!

Juice: As most juices have a lot of sugar I minimize it. 1 cup a day at best, as calories are high. If you use 24 oz. of juice in the evening shake you may be hungry afterwards. Use caution. As juices taste good there is no need to enhance the flavor, however, what I often do, especially in the summer, is mix 2-3 oz. of juice with 10-12 oz. of flavored mineral water for a great tasting, very refreshing drink- with ice, and very few calories!

Shakes: I prefer powder based diet shakes and I add the no/low calorie flavorings I mentioned in Chapter 1 to make them taste good. Walk through your grocery store aisles and you will find numerous products that will make these shakes taste very good and provide the refreshment and nourishment you need. I do recommend vitamins and minerals with the evening shake- again, contact me if you want to know what shake mixes and supplements I recommend. Add ice cubes or ice slivers- maybe even a little fruit- and these drinks or shakes can be as tasty as many ice cream dishes, yet they help you lose weight and fill you up- for a long time.

Soda: I suggest diet, with no caffeine. 1-2 per day maximum in place of water, if you prefer.

Meat, poultry, fish: no need for bread or a sandwich, unless it is real/true whole wheat or grain bread. Just the meats seasoned as you like, is my recommendation. Avoid too much salt, but look at the seasonings you can add, or condiments, to make a fair amount of high protein food taste very, very good- without starchy breads! After your liquids, a nice serving of high protein food will fill you up!

Eggs: I like them any way I can get them. 6 per week is about my maximum. Hard boiled or deviled eggs are great late night snacks- if you are truly hungry! Don't be surprised if you are not.

Vegetables: again, walk through any grocery store and look at the countless ways to season and flavor vegetables so they taste good! Often, I will have 16 oz. of the vegetable(s) of my choice seasoned with a little parmesan cheese, garlic, onion, pepper, or related seasonings, perhaps butter or similar substitute, and I have had a lot of food that tastes great and fills me up. I do prefer high protein foods, though.

Fruit: 1 piece a day, is all I recommend during weight loss. Any kind.

Nuts: I like all. Minimal or no salt is suggested.

Fats: butter and some dairy products, like skim milk. Be careful- keep the fat and calorie content down!

The key is to shop for seasonings and flavorings that will make your water, shakes, creative liquids and fluids, foods, meats, etc. taste great while you lose weight, while you also don't feel hungry. Most of the foods I suggest you avoid are processed.

No surprise, yet my food budget- (cost)- is <u>less</u> with the daily water, liquid and food intake I have identified. Lose weight, look great, feel great, spend less- sound good? (Read Chapter 4, but then we get really specific in Chapter 5 on Great tasting water, liquids and foods that help you lose weight!)

CHAPTER 4

What about my

energy?

As I have mentioned, mine is fine and I have a demanding job and my hobby, which I will soon explain, demands a lot of energy. My body- and yours- needs a lot of water, adequate vitamins and minerals, lean meats, poultry and fish, and vegetables. Add a little fruit and nuts and you have a full diet of good tasting foods and liquids that will help you lose weight- without noticing it! Energy is of no concern to me and, again, I do not use caffeine, ephedra or any other stimulants- and haven't for 22 years. The food and liquid intake I have identified gives me all the energy I need. I add, I avoid/minimize sugar and salt.

Experiment if you wish, but the regimen I have outlined, with a lot of latitude for your particular needs, works. I am no different than you. There is more than enough energy available for the most demanding schedules, and a great night's sleep is had as well. I think we've covered this subject pretty thoroughly- you'll read how I can prove it, soon.

CHAPTER 5
What VERY specific ingredients can make water, shakes and low calorie foods taste GREAT!

(I know this is a bit repetitious but you want your water, drinks, shakes and food to taste great- right?)

Liquids: I prefer flavored mineral water as it tastes great chilled, on ice, and is very refreshing. Or, tap or distilled water- chilled or on ice, with a slice of lemon, lime or orange is great, too. Often, I will mix 2-3 oz. of fruit juice or lemonade with 10-12 oz. of flavored mineral water for a drink I really love- especially on warm days. Add ice to quench your thirst.

Diet drinks- sodas, or fruity tasting low calorie drinks- are OK in moderation as an occasional substitute for water. Regular fruit juices have a lot of sugar, often, and should be used very sparingly. For a warm drink, bouillon cubes, in any flavor, provide a broth-like drink that is, primarily water, yet tastes very good. Have 8-16 oz. and your calorie intake is very low; but watch the sodium content of broth(s)! If you need to chill your palate, lime or lemon juice, added to icy water can liven the flavor- especially with, what else, ice.

Shakes: diet, or powdered, drinks are recommended, especially for the evening meal.

Flavors like chocolate, vanilla, strawberry, etc. are all available. (For the brand I recommend please contact me- or shop for what you are familiar with or whatever strikes your fancy). 2 scoops of powder are enough. Add skim milk, and water - about 16 to 24 oz. of each, then ice, and add fat free pudding mix (1-2 tablespoons), maybe a piece of fruit (banana, orange), or berries to sweeten the flavor. Lite ice cream- one small scoop- adds flavor. Ice cream toppings- lite- in small amounts, can add a lot of flavor. I like fat-free pudding mixes, 1-2 tablespoons per shake: chocolate, banana cream, vanilla, pistachio, butterscotch, etc. A couple squirts of honey can add a nice sweet flavor, also. Maybe a little fat or sugar free whipped cream; natural apple or fruit sauces, non-sugar sweeteners, etc. can all make a powdered, milk based drink taste great. Don't forget the ice to give you 64 oz.! Your stomach will be quite full!

Fruit based shakes- not my favorite, but some people prefer them. Use 8-16 oz. of fruit juices or drinks, the powder or liquid diet drink ingredients, and other fruit flavors. But add water and ice. Perhaps some no/low calorie fruity drinks- which will usually contain artificial sweeteners- will enhance the flavor with very few calories. Add some real fruit or berries- sweeten to taste. But watch the calories and the amount of sugar!! I don't recommend fruit based drinks unless you prefer them or need to use them.

Food Based Flavorings: a walk down the grocery aisle will display a plethora of options to make any vegetable, or lean meat, tasted superb. Here are just a few (well, maybe a bit more):

Fat free/low cal/low carb salad dressings. Condiments like: relishes, mustard, ketchup, etc. Soy sauce. Salsa(s). Worcestershire, Tobasco, Hot sauces, etc. Pickles- as additions to vegetable servings or alone. Steak Sauces- low cal. Vinegar based dressings. Sweet/sour toppings. Salad toppings (the kinds in jars). Grated low-cal cheese. Tomato sauces and derivatives. Spices- dozens to choose from. Butter or margarine substitutes. Lite sour cream.

For a fruitier taste, try <u>natural</u> apple or fruit sauces or sugar free/low sugar jellies, jam or even honey.

KEY: shop for flavorings that will taste good <u>and</u> be low in calories. There are hundreds to choose from! Who says vegetables and lean meats can't taste great and be low in calories?

CHAPTER 6

For men it's twelve but eleven for ladies

For those who like or want to count calories here is a simple formula to follow:

It seems, for men, we can consume 12 times our ideal body weight, in calories, and we will reach, or maintain that weight. If a man wants to weigh 200#, then, 2400 calories per day, (200 x 12), may maintain that weight. For women though, it seems the magic multiplier is 11. So, if a lady wants to achieve or maintain a weight of 150#, then, she could consume 1650, (150 x 11), calories per day and she would probably reach or keep her weight around 150#. The reason men seem to be able to consume 12 times their body weight, is perhaps due to a faster metabolism most men seem to have. It is very easy to keep track of calories with this simple formula, if you want to. But, if you follow the liquid/water/diet drink/high protein and vegetable program already identified, you won't need to- and you will probably not want much food as you'll be full and have plenty of energy. Now, let's get to the fun part.........

CHAPTER 7

MYB= Move Your Body

If you are keeping track of calories coming in, as in Chapter 6, here is an easy way to keep track of calories going "out".

If a person walks or runs 1 mile, a 150 pound person will "burn" 100 calories. If a 200 pound person walks or runs 1 mile they will burn 133 calories. The formula is:

Your weight divided by 150 = calories "burned" per mile, or

<u>Your weight</u>
150
equals calories burned per mile.

Whether you walk, jog or run, are male or female, it doesn't matter- a 150# pound person "burns" about 100 calories per mile whether walking, jogging or running. So, if a 200 pound man can consume 2400 calories and maintain his weight, if he walks or runs 3 miles a day his "net" calorie intake is 2001. (2400 calories of food and liquids, minus 399 calories of walking - 3 miles at 133 calories burned per mile- totals 2001 net calories- less than he needs to weigh 200#; 2400-399 = 2001). So, what happens? He loses weight with minimal effort! And, if he will follow the liquid and food intake program previously identified there aren't 2400 calories in that combination! Result, further weight loss. Lose 50 pounds in 50 days? Yes, I did it and still weigh what I did in 1990 at age 35, which I also weighed at age 20. It works!

For a lady, then, if her desired weight was 150# she can consume about 1650 calories per day; if she walks, jogs or runs 3 miles she will have burned off about 300 calories- (remember: a 150# person expends 100 calories, approximately, for every mile). She, then would have 1350 "net" calories for the day (1650 − 300 = 1350)- same as for our male example, she will lose weight. Also, there are not 1650 calories in the liquid and food intake program identified. Which means: more weight loss!

But, I don't have time to walk 3 miles. Or, I don't like- or can't- jog or run. Or, I like other activities, but not exercise. Then, consider these options:

<u>The Hidden Mile (or two)</u>:

The average person walks a mile in 15-20 minutes. Before going off to work or school, walk 5 to 20 minutes. Do the same at mid day. On your lunch break, walk 10-30 minutes. Add it up. That's 1-2 miles, minimum. At a leisurely pace. Yes, you do have time. Add a mile in the evening and you have 3. Walk more if you like it or want more rapid weight loss. Watch your energy improve and tell your body it wants more walking. My point is whenever you have 5, or more, minutes- on a break, while waiting, at lunch, in the evening, walk at a comfortable pace. Your body does not know if you are walking while on a work break, during a lunch period, while you are waiting for kids to finish an activity, while you are waiting for a ride, in an airport, in a hotel, outdoors, in a mall, during an intermission, etc. None of those things matter- just Move Your Body! You will lose weight faster, with leisurely walking, and watch your mood improve as you walk and get your blood circulating. For runners and joggers, it only takes 20-30 minutes to go 3 miles.

Do this every day- walk, jog, or run; consume the liquids and discretionary foods identified; watch calories if you like, and, guess what? You will lose weight- as this basic regime will help you lose weight, modify it or maintain it to keep your weight where you want it. We all have the Hidden Mile, or two, or three in our daily routines. If some days only allow 1-2 miles, make up the deficit the next day- or on the weekend. We all have 1-2 hours of time to walk and Move Our Bodies on the weekend. For golfers, this is easy. Don't use the cart!

But, what about other activities if I can't jog, walk or run- or don't like those?

I don't know anyone who does not like to walk 5-10 minutes a few times a day. But for those people who prefer biking, tennis, racquet sports, basketball, weight training, aerobic training, swimming, martial arts, etc,:

For me, I have to bike 3-4 miles to feel I have burned as many calories as one mile of walking or jogging. That seems to be common- for many, biking is easier. Swimming seems comparable to running in terms of calorie expenditure. Racquet sports, tennis, and basketball seem to equate to jogging or running in terms of calories used and energy spent. Consider, and keep track of, the actual time you are "active" (moving) in any of these activities and determine how many minutes you have utilized. Try to equate that to 1 mile of walking, jogging or running- you'll develop a "feel" to measure your "Move Your Body" activity, and potential calories burned. I have been lifting weights for 33 years, at the time of this writing, and that activity, for me, does not burn as many calories as walking or jogging. About half as many, in my view. However, lifting weights with little, or no time, between sets can be a way to increase calorie consumption as your body is moving faster and working harder- circuit type training, but with weights that allow no more than 6 repetitions, then on to the next set. The best exercise I have ever experienced is a rigorous hour of martial arts training. 2-4 hours a week is <u>plenty.</u>

Gardening, mowing the lawn, housecleaning, garage/lawn work, etc. are other forms of Moving Your Body- keep track of what you have done in a given day and equate it to how far you may have walked. You'll find a way to convert any Move Your Body activity into calorie consumption, in a way you can fairly measure.

So, how do I Move My Body? I walk 6-10 miles per week. I jog 6-8 miles per week (I want 12-18 miles per week as my goal, combined). I lift weights twice a week. Total time spent: 6-8 hours per week; 4-5 during the week, 2-3 on weekends. I improve and maintain my weight and health in the process. I am competing in martial arts again, and power lifting- after a 20 year sabbatical. I have won 5 trophies during the past 6 months. I will be 50 in January of 2005. Moving Your Body maintains your body's strength and vitality. I also follow the liquid regimen I identified in the beginning. I like good tasting mineral water, flavored tap or distilled water and diet/powder shakes; and my food bill is much less than most people spend. Much less.

CHAPTER 8
Chart your progress

It is important to keep track of what you put into your body, and what you expend from it. I strongly recommend you weigh yourself daily. Late afternoon is best for me, before my evening shake, or try mornings if you prefer.

Keep track of how you are Moving Your Body-miles, approximate miles, minutes or hours spent in a given activity, etc. It only takes a moment a few times day to do this:

(Contact me for a companion notebook like this to keep track of your daily progress)

DAY _____

Weight _____

Liquids consumed: (describe)

Morning_____

Mid-day_____

Lunch_____

Afternoon_____

Evening_____

Foods consumed: (describe)

(*Stop, and ask yourself: do I really need food, at this point, after my liquids?) If I still do, I ate:*

Morning_____

_____

Lunch_____

_____

Dinner_____

_____

Other (snacks)

_____

_____

Moving My Body today- I did the following:

Walked _____miles

Jogged/Ran _____miles

Biked _____miles

Other Activities

_____

_____

_____

If I were to calculate the calories I expended walking, jogging or running; or equate these "other activities" into miles walked, or minutes/ hours spent, about how many calories do I feel I "burned' today:

_____

(Math: 1 mile for a 150# person = approximately 100 calories burned. Your weight, divided by 150, will equal about how many calories you burn walking, jogging or running 1 mile; therefore, a 200 pound person burns about 133 calories per mile, a 250 pound person burns about 167 per mile, or a 300 pound person burns about 200 per mile.)

Then, subtract the calories you spent Moving Your Body from the calories you consumed and you have a "net" calorie deficit or excess. Remember: deficits are good as they will mean weight loss. If you have an occasional "excess" day, be a bit more careful or Move Your Body a bit more the next few days to compensate. It works.

Calories I consumed today_____

Calories I "spent" Moving My Body_____

My Net Calorie Deficit today is _____or, excess is _____

Note: for a daily work book to keep track of the above information please contact me at sspribyl@new.rr.com.

CHAPTER 9

Control your

Surroundings!

Take a look in your refrigerator, food shelves and pantry. If you have foods that don't meet the ones I propose to you throw them out, give them to charity or friends, etc. When you shop, only buy 1 week's worth of food at a time- and buy the right foods! If "bad" foods are not in your home, how can you eat them? If you only have "good" liquids and foods, that taste wonderful, and are all you have to choose from, that is all you will eat. If you desire snacks- which is doubtful if you follow the 100+ oz. of daily liquid consumption, with a bit of appropriate food if you are really hungry, you will lose weight. "Moving Your Body" as much as you can or want will accelerate your weight loss. (I've identified several foods and liquid drinks and shakes; and, by all means, search your grocery store for creative ways to drink and eat foods that help you lose weight, taste fantastic, are good for you, cost little, help you look the way you want, wear the clothes you want, etc.)

When you dine out, by now, you know what to look for: salads with no/low fat dressings, lean cuts of meat, poultry, or fish (not fried!), vegetables instead of potatoes of any sort!, vegetable or meat broth based soup instead of bread, avoid desserts. (If you splurge, or make a mistake, the next day..... walk an extra 2 miles to compensate!)

Chapter 10

A New, Permanent you with a little help

In this book I have identified ways that I have proven, for almost 15 years, will help you lose weight. For me, 50 pounds in 50 days. Why not for you? I am no different than you.

Once you attain your goal weight, I suggest you back off the liquid intake to about 64 to 80 oz. per day, from 100+, but still drink the same liquids as your body will crave them! Eat more vegetables, fruit, whole grain bread, nuts and lean meats, poultry, and fish. But you must continue to weigh yourself daily! If you gain a pound, you now know how to get rid of it! This is a permanent technique you have learned. But only you can use discipline yourself to use it. So,

Regardless your religious or spiritual beliefs, I strongly recommend 10-40 minutes per day be spent in silent prayer or meditation. Reflect on the many blessings you have received and the many gifts you have to offer others. Then, again silently, ask your creator, or inner self, to guide you to the weight you know you were naturally born to weigh at this point in your life. I have given you the recipe. Your creator, or inner self that knows everything about you, will give you the guidance and strength to lose the weight you want, look the way you naturally should and you may just find you have learned much more than just weight loss. The new you will be more than just the person you are so happy to see in the mirror. The time to start your new journey is now. Thank you, and may your goals, dreams and potential all be realized.

www.ingramcontent.com/pod-product-compliance
Lightning Source LLC
Chambersburg PA
CBHW020353290526
45785CB00005B/2261